Essential Oils

30 Recipes To Help You Look Younger

Table of content

Introduction

You get online and look up recipes for certain foods you ought to be eating. There are lists as long as the empire state building is tall, and you have no idea how you are going to get them all into your diet.

If only there was a concentrated form of the plant you could use to get the same benefits, but in less time and with less product.

You read the ingredient label on the stress medication, or you look into aroma therapy, and what you find is another list of long ingredients, many of which you can't pronounce. You don't like to put all of that stuff into or on your body, but you don't want to have those wrinkles or feel that stress, either.

So what do you do? There has got to be a way you can treat your aging skin with natural ingredients that actually work, or there has to be a natural way to deal with the stress in your life, that doesn't require you to turn into a zombie in the process.

As a matter of fact, there is. Essential oils are the concentrated form of all the things you know that are good for you and will help you stay young. When you are able to use these oils in your day, you are using things that will keep your skin bright and fresh, fade those wrinkles, and make that stress go away.

There is no end to the ways you can use oils to benefit your day. Whether you like to use them topically, or if you would rather heat them in a warmer, you are going to get the insane benefits that come with each oil.

And what makes this even better is that you can combine the oils and get the best of both! Use two or three at a time to treat a variety of illnesses, ailments, or conditions you want to go away.

With this guide to help you, you will find an oil for everything you could imagine.

Want better hair? Got it. Want better skin? Got it. Want fewer wrinkles? Gone. What about less stress in your day?

There's an oil for that, too.

It won't take long before you realize these oils are your best friend, and your solution to a variety of problems. Get ready to take a new spin on life, and you will never go back to those chemical filled treatments again.

Chapter 1 – A Brief History on Essential Oils

We all know that oils have been around for a long time, but that is pretty vague if you want to know the actual history behind the oils. Let's take a second before we get into the use of the oils and learn where they came from originally, and what they have been used for in the past.

As a whole, essential oils have also gone by the name aroma oils as that is how they were most often used. Even in ancient times, people would heat the oil to release the fragrance and enjoy the beneficial properties that came from the oils.

Across the globe, the use of the oils ranged from religious use to medicinal. It wasn't until quite recently that many people started using for recreational purposes.

Egypt

While we can go across the planet and see evidence of many different tribes using oils for a variety of different things, we can pinpoint the Egyptians as the earliest people that used essential oils with any form of regularity. They used all kinds for a variety of reasons, from funeral rituals to wedding feasts and everything in between.

It is interesting to note, however that only the Egyptian priests were allowed to use the oils in any ceremony, because they believed the powers of the oils to be sacred, and thus forbid anyone that wasn't close to their gods to use the oils in any way.

Research has shown that they dedicated certain fragrances to specific deity, and would use the specific oils on their leaders as they prepared them for mummification.

Even with this tight stipulation, however, the people as a whole still largely enjoyed the use of all kinds of oils in their day to day lives.

The Orient and Europe

Egypt wasn't alone, however, in their use of oil through time. China and the other countries of the Far East are also recorded to use them in a variety of ways. They would use them in their own spiritual rituals, but they focused more on the healing benefits they found in the oils than they did in the spiritual aspect.

France has had its share of oil popularity, and so have the other European countries as well. As you can see this is a practice that is world renowned.

Chapter 2 – Oils for Skin and Beauty

No matter how old you are, there is something you wish you could do with your skin. Something that would make it feel better, something that would make it look younger, something that would make it healthier.

Now, you can do all three of those things with these oils. You can use each one as is, or you can mix in your lotion to get the benefits of the oil after you are done in the shower or before you start your day. When you use these oils, you are going to see a youthful shine in your skin you didn't notice was there before, and you will fall in love with the results.

There is no way you will ever go back to the other way you were taking care of your skin again. Say hello to beauty, and goodbye to spending all of that money on products that don't give you the results they say they do.

This is your dream come true for your skin care regime, and all you have to do is blend a few oils. Life just got a whole lot easier, and your new, beautiful self is about to take the stage and flaunt what you got.

Carrot Seed Frankincense Revitalizer

10 drops carrot seed oil

10 drops frankincense oil

Mix the oils together and store in an oil jar. When you are ready to use them, blend in a carrier oil to minimize the irritation on your skin.

Carrot seed oil is the perfect oil for reducing scars, and frankincense is well known for its moisturizing capabilities... no more wrinkles!

Tea Tree Delight

10 drops tee tree oil

5 drops lemon oil

5 drops lavender oil

Mix the oils together and store in an oil jar. When you are ready to use them, blend in a carrier oil to minimize the irritation on your skin.

Lavender oil is going to make your skin soft and silky, while the tea tree clears up any blemish you want gone!

The Acne Buster

15 drops geranium oil

10 drops tea tree oil

Mix the oils together and store in an oil jar. When you are ready to use them, blend in a carrier oil to minimize the irritation on your skin.

Acne won't stand a chance when you use this combination in the morning!

The Three Wisemen Blend

10 drops frankincense

10 drops myrrh

5 drops goldenrod

Mix the oils together and store in an oil jar. When you are ready to use them, blend in a carrier oil to minimize the irritation on your skin.

You couldn't ask for a better combination to reduce the appearance of fine lines and wrinkles. Say hello to smooth skin once again!

Sunny Rose Blend

15 drops rose oil

10 drops lemon oil

Mix the oils together and store in an oil jar. When you are ready to use them, blend in a carrier oil to minimize the irritation on your skin.

Rose oil is the perfect thing to get rid of age spots or wrinkles, and when paired with lemon, it is unstoppable.

Neroli Clean

15 drops neroli

10 drops tea tree

Mix the oils together and store in an oil jar. When you are ready to use them, blend in a carrier oil to minimize the irritation on your skin.

You couldn't ask for a better blend when you are trying to fight age or signs of aging or acne!

Garden Fairy Blend

15 drops lavender

15 drops rosewood

Mix the oils together and store in an oil jar. When you are ready to use them, blend in a carrier oil to minimize the irritation on your skin.

Rose oil is great for helping with acne, and lavender will get rid of the dry patches. You can create your own blend for moisture and clear skin with this.

Patchouli Parade

10 drops patchouli

10 drops tea tree

Mix the oils together and store in an oil jar. When you are ready to use them, blend in a carrier oil to minimize the irritation on your skin.

Patchouli takes care of dryness and oiliness both, it is like the best acne moisturizer on the planet, but it's entirely natural!

The Ylang Ylang Yin Yang

Mix the oils together and store in an oil jar. When you are ready to use them, blend in a carrier oil to minimize the irritation on your skin.

20 drops ylang ylang

20 drops frankincense

Frankincense and ylang ylang both restore the elasticity in your skin. If you want to reduce wrinkles, this is your perfectly balanced pair.

Total Package Power

5 drops ylang ylang

5 drops tea tree

5 drops lavender

5 drops myrrh

Mix the oils together and store in an oil jar. When you are ready to use them, blend in a carrier oil to minimize the irritation on your skin.

Anything you want done to your skin, this is going to do. Whether you want your skin to have fewer wrinkles, your acne to disappear, or to take care of those dry patches, you will have it when you use this oil.

Chapter 3 – Oils to Reduce Stress

Let's face it, we would like to think that our job is more stressful than any other job on the planet, but that is just not the case. Everyone has a life full of stress, and in our fast paced society, stress is taking root in ways it never has before. Funny as it sounds, stress isn't new to the world, and neither are the ways to treat it.

There are all kinds of natural methods people can use to reduce the stress in their life, but few of them are as beneficial as using essential oils. You can blend the oils that you like the best, and have that perfect dream scent greet you as you settle into a nice hot bath, or you can blend a number of the oils for your perfect scent sensation.

Even if you only want to use one of the oils in a recipe, that's fine, too! You need to do what you want to make your happy and get the most out of your essential oil experience. That is what they are there for, and that is what I want to teach you how to do with this book.

All too often you are told you can do it wrong, but I want you to rest assured you can't with this, and gain the confidence you need to make your essential bliss.

Bergamot Diffuser

10 drops bergamot

10 drops lavender

If you would like to burn this instead, place 5 drops in your oil warmer with a bit of water, if you want it diluted.

Bergamot has a strong fragrance, and when breathed in, it is known to reduce stress instantly.

Marjoram Jam

10 drops marjoram

10 drops bergamot

Mix the oils together and store in an oil jar. When you are ready to use them, blend in a carrier oil to minimize the irritation on your skin.

If you would rather use in a warmer or a diffuser, add 5 drops to the warmer directly and use a tea light to heat it.

This is the perfect blend to reduce anxiety and calm any mental pain you feel.

Vetiver Reviver

15 drops vetiver

5 drops tea tree

5 drops lavender

Mix the oils together and store in an oil jar. When you are ready to use them, blend in a carrier oil to minimize the irritation on your skin.

If you would rather use in a warmer or a diffuser, add 5 drops to the warmer directly and use a tea light to heat it.

Have you ever wanted to face the day like a brand new challenge? That is exactly what these oils will do for you!

The Clear Mind Potion

10 drops lemon

10 drops chamomile

Mix the oils together and store in an oil jar. When you are ready to use them, blend in a carrier oil to minimize the irritation on your skin.

If you would rather use in a warmer or a diffuser, add 5 drops to the warmer directly and use a tea light to heat it.

Breathe this blend in deeply for clarity of the mind and soul.

Geranium Pick-me-up

10 drops geranium

10 drops lemon

Mix the oils together and store in an oil jar. When you are ready to use them, blend in a carrier oil to minimize the irritation on your skin.

If you would rather use in a warmer or a diffuser, add 5 drops to the warmer directly and use a tea light to heat it.

Geranium is the one oil that is known to pick up down moods, making everything feel all right once again!

A Fennel Funnel

10 drops fennel

10 drops rose

5 drops geranium

Mix the oils together and store in an oil jar. When you are ready to use them, blend in a carrier oil to minimize the irritation on your skin.

If you would rather use in a warmer or a diffuser, add 5 drops to the warmer directly and use a tea light to heat it.

This oil will make you feel vibrant and alive, helping you help yourself.

Ylang Ylang Cinnamon Bear

10 drops cinnamon

10 drops ylang ylang

5 drops orange

Mix the oils together and store in an oil jar. When you are ready to use them, blend in a carrier oil to minimize the irritation on your skin.

If you would rather use in a warmer or a diffuser, add 5 drops to the warmer directly and use a tea light to heat it.

The sweet spice of this fragrance will help you reduce that frustration and keep your cool under the harshest circumstances.

Lavender Laughter

10 drops lavender

10 drops myrrh

Mix the oils together and store in an oil jar. When you are ready to use them, blend in a carrier oil to minimize the irritation on your skin.

If you would rather use in a warmer or a diffuser, add 5 drops to the warmer directly and use a tea light to heat it.

If you ever want to feel relaxed and lifted, try this blend in your diffuser.

A Walk Among Roses

10 drops rose oil

5 drops cinnamon

Mix the oils together and store in an oil jar. When you are ready to use them, blend in a carrier oil to minimize the irritation on your skin.

If you would rather use in a warmer or a diffuser, add 5 drops to the warmer directly and use a tea light to heat it.

Try this blend if you want to feel the wonders of the outdoors, but you don't want to leave your house.

Sunshine on my Shoulders

15 drops goldenseal

10 drops cedar

10 drops lemon

Mix the oils together and store in an oil jar. When you are ready to use them, blend in a carrier oil to minimize the irritation on your skin.

If you would rather use in a warmer or a diffuser, add 5 drops to the warmer directly and use a tea light to heat it.

This is a nice, mountain like fragrance that will carry you away on the hills of your dreams.

Queen of Roses

10 drops rose oil

10 drops rosewood oil

Mix the oils together and store in an oil jar. When you are ready to use them, blend in a carrier oil to minimize the irritation on your skin.

If you would rather use in a warmer or a diffuser, add 5 drops to the warmer directly and use a tea light to heat it.

This is a very floral blend that will clear your mind and help you relax even after the most hectic of days.

Chapter 4 – Healing Oils and Other Combinations

Looking younger, becoming healthier, and reducing the stress in your life are several main reasons you would want to use essential oils, but did you know there are other reasons you can use them?

In this chapter, I am going to show you the other things you can do with essential oils, and how you can mix them even more to get more benefits out of it. I want you to be the best you can be, and when you are able to use these all in different combinations, the benefits are so abundant you won't have to use more than a couple of blends a day.

Have fun with these, and use the ideas to blend your own oils. You can mix and match as you please to get the custom oil that is perfect for your own situation. Nothing gets more custom than that, and you will have the essential oil you need for anything that you want.

It couldn't get any better than that.

Citrus Burst

10 drops lemon

10 drops orange

10 drops red orange

Mix the oils together and store in an oil jar. When you are ready to use them, blend in a carrier oil to minimize the irritation on your skin.

Kick any cold to the curb with this blend of the warmest citrus oils.

Peppermint Paddy

10 drops peppermint

5 drops lemongrass

Mix the oils together and store in an oil jar. When you are ready to use them, blend in a carrier oil to minimize the irritation on your skin.

A charming scent to clear your house of any ill will and bring in the sunshine you crave.

Skipping Through the Woods

10 drops cedar oil

5 drops wood blend

5 drops pine

1 drop tea tree oil

Mix the oils together and store in an oil jar. When you are ready to use them, blend in a carrier oil to minimize the irritation on your skin.

Warm this oil if you ever have a headache that needs attention, and you won't have to reach for those pain killers ever again.

Holiday All the Year Round

10 drops cinnamon oil

5 drops peppermint

Mix the oils together and store in an oil jar. When you are ready to use them, blend in a carrier oil to minimize the irritation on your skin.

Warm this oil if you want to bring in a burst of that holiday cheer any time of the year. Whether you want to make it warm and cozy or if you want to just grab that bit of Christmas cheer, this is the scent for you!

Mint Madness

10 drops peppermint

10 drops spearmint

Mix the oils together and store in an oil jar. When you are ready to use them, blend in a carrier oil to minimize the irritation on your skin.

Use this oil across your forehead for instant relief from a headache, or across your tummy to reduce stomach pain.

Scar Remover Deluxe

6 drops patchouli

6 drops peppermint

6 drops lavender

Mix the oils together and store in an oil jar. When you are ready to use them, blend in a carrier oil to minimize the irritation on your skin.

Apply several times throughout the day, and watch that scar disappear right before your eyes.

Happy Hearts

5 drops sunflower oil

5 drops argon

5 drops lemon

Mix the oils together and store in an oil jar. When you are ready to use them, blend in a carrier oil to minimize the irritation on your skin.

Place a dab behind each ear for a day filled with fun and stress free laughter. You can also put this in your diffuser if you want to make a scent that will bring cheerfulness to anyone that enters your home.

Dust Buster 5000

10 drops orange

10 drops cinnamon

10 drops lemon

Mix the oils together and store in an oil jar. When you are ready to use them, spray on a cleaning cloth and use to wipe up any counter space or floor space you want to have a little bit of extra attention. There's no way you can miss a thing when you are using this cleaning blend of oils.

Just a Dandy Diddy

10 drops sunflower oil

5 drops saffron oil

6 drops lavender oil

Mix the oils together and store in an oil jar. When you are ready to use them, blend in a carrier oil to minimize the irritation on your skin.

This is a great oil to rub on your hands for extra moisture that lotion just can't seem to reach, and you can use it under your nose when you have a cold to reduce stuffiness and pain from blowing your nose all the time.

Drops of Cheerfulness

10 drops peppermint

10 drops lavender

10 drops fennel

Mix the oils together and store in an oil jar. When you are ready to use them, blend in a carrier oil to minimize the irritation on your skin.

If you would like to burn this instead, place 5 drops in your oil warmer with a bit of water, if you want it diluted.

Chapter 5 – How to Use Essential Oils Effectively

If you look online, it won't take you long before you are bombarded with all kinds of conflicting opinions when it comes to the use of essential oils. There are those that say you need to stick with a specific brand. There are those that say you can ingest them. There are those that tell you to never ingest them for any reason.

At the end of the day, it is important for you to do what works for you, and not to be swayed with the general opinion of the population. If that means you stick with one single brand for your oils, go for it, but if you want to explore and use varying brands for different oils, that's just fine, too.

You really can't do it wrong, you just have to learn what you want and go with that. Of course, you will find that there are brands that like to bundle oils and orders to help you save money, but that really doesn't have any bearing on how the oils work.

How do I use my oils?

Are they safe to ingest?

Although it doesn't matter what brand you use for your oils, how you use your oils does matter.

For starters, ingesting oils is a very controversial topic and it is best left up to you what you would like to do with your oils, however, it is important to note that while some people may feel comfortable ingesting them, all oils are toxic when taken in high amounts and you should never take more than a drop in heavily diluted water.

More is not better!

Stick to the lesser amount and you will still get the benefits you want.

Can I apply them directly to my skin?

Again, this is dependent on the particular oil you are using. Some oils, such as basil oil, is so strong it will burn you if it is applied directly to your skin. If you are going to use the oils topically, you need to read to find which ones are safe to apply to your skin directly, and which ones you have to only use for aroma therapy.

If you are going to use oil on your skin directly, it is a good idea to use a carrier oil to alleviate any potential burns you may get from that oil on your skin. A carrier oil is an oil that is fine on your skin no matter where you put it, and there are a whole list of carrier oils that are fine to use in combination with any other oil.

The carrier oil I recommend the most is coconut oil. It is good for your skin, which puts it above the other carrier oils that do nothing for your skin, it's easy to get, and it isn't going to interfere with any of the oils you are using for your health.

What about this aroma therapy method?

Probably the most popular method, aroma therapy has a wide range of benefits. Not only are you going to get the same benefits you would from the oil if you were to apply it directly, but you are going to be rewarded with a delicious smell through your house.

There is a reason this was one of the most popular methods of using the oil, and remains so to this day. It is safe for your skin, it gives you the same benefits as ingesting does, and it makes your house smell good.

An all-around win for anyone that wants to use oils.

How do I go about using the oils in aroma therapy?

Simply use an oil warmer, they are easy to find in store or second hand. And they may come electric or with tea light candles. Simply place a couple of drops in the warmer and warm.

You can dilute with water if you like, but that isn't necessary for the use of the oil so you can really do what you want with that one. Just make sure you keep your warmer under supervision as you don't want a pet or a child to accidently knock it over with the hot oil inside.

When the oil is heated, it is going to release a wonderful fragrance into the air for you to breathe in. Breathe in deeply when you are near the warmer for the full effect, or stay in the room while the oil is burning to go about your day. You will get the same benefits either way, but breathing them in deliberately is going to get you the results a lot faster than if you were to light the oil and leave it while you went about your day.

I hope you enjoyed this book and everything you can do with essential oils, and I know you will fall in love with the benefits as soon as you start. They come quickly, so you don't have to wait very long before you see exactly what you were hoping for with these oils.

Conclusion

There you have it, everything you need to know to look younger and feel better the natural way, with essential oils you have on hand. It won't take long before you realize these oils are good for everything, and you can use them for nearly any ailment you see.

They are small, non-invasive, and easy to use, so why would you go through the painful process of going to the store, standing in line, and spending hours trying to decide which product is right for you when you know the descriptions are just designed to get you to buy that product anyway?

When you jump into the world of oil, you will open the door to doing life the healthy way. No more stress, no more mess, and no more wondering what the next product will be to hopefully help you out.

Use these oils with confidence that you will feel better, look better, and be better. They have been in use for centuries for a reason, and they aren't about to fail on you now.

So what are you waiting for?

You have oils to mix.

FREE Bonus Reminder

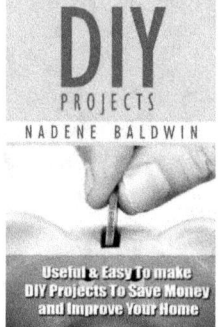

If you have not grabbed it yet, please go ahead and download your special bonus report *"DIY Projects. 13 Useful & Easy To Make DIY Projects To Save Money & Improve Your Home!"*

Simply Click the Button Below

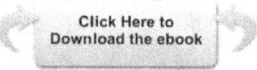

OR **Go to This Page**

http://diyhomecraft.com/free

BONUS #2: More Free & Discounted Books

Do you want to receive more Free & Discounted Books?

We have a mailing list where we send out our new Books when they go free or with a discount on Kindle. Click on the link below to sign up for Free & Discount Book Promotions.

=> Sign Up for Free & Discount Book Promotions <=

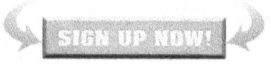

OR Go to this URL

http://zbit.ly/1WBb1Ek

www.ingramcontent.com/pod-product-compliance
Lightning Source LLC
Chambersburg PA
CBHW061951280526
45787CB00004B/1817

* 9 7 8 1 5 4 8 0 5 8 6 4 7 *